ARTHRITIS

DIET

COOKBOOK

GEORGE ANDERSON

INTRODUCTION

Arthritis

Arthritis is a term often used to mean any disorder that affects joints. Symptoms generally include joint pain and stiffness. Other symptoms may include redness, warmth, swelling, and decreased range of motion of the affected joints. In some types of arthritis, other organs are also affected. Onset can be gradual or sudden.

There are over 100 types of arthritis. The most common forms are osteoarthritis (degenerative joint disease) and rheumatoid arthritis. Osteoarthritis usually occurs with age and affects the fingers, knees, and hips. Rheumatoid arthritis is an autoimmune disorder that often affects the hands and feet. Other types include gout, lupus, fibromyalgia, and septic arthritis. They are all types of rheumatic disease.

Treatment may include resting the joint and alternating between applying ice and heat. Weight loss and exercise may also be useful. Recommended medications may depend on the form of arthritis. These may include pain medications such as ibuprofen and paracetamol (acetaminophen). In some circumstances, a joint replacement may be useful.

Osteoarthritis affects more than 3.8% of people, while rheumatoid arthritis affects about 0.24% of people. Gout affects about 1–2% of the Western population at some point in their lives. In Australia about 15% of people are affected by arthritis, while in the United States more than 20% have a type of arthritis. Overall the disease becomes more common with age. Arthritis is a common reason that people miss work and can result in a decreased quality of life. The term is derived from arthr- (meaning 'joint') and (meaning 'inflammation').

Classification of arthritis

There are several diseases where joint pain is primary, and is considered the main feature. Generally when a person has "arthritis" it means that they have one of these diseases, which include:

- Osteoarthritis

- Rheumatoid arthritis

- Gout and pseudo-gout

- Septic arthritis

- Ankylosing spondylitis

- Juvenile idiopathic arthritis

- Still's disease

- Psoriatic arthritis

Joint pain can also be a symptom of other diseases. In this case, the arthritis is considered to be secondary to the main disease; these include:

- Psoriasis

- Reactive arthritis

- Ehlers–Danlos syndrome

- Iron overload

- Hepatitis

- Lyme disease

- Sjögren's disease

- Hashimoto's thyroiditis

- Celiac disease

- Non-celiac gluten sensitivity

- Inflammatory bowel disease (including Crohn's disease and ulcerative colitis)

- Henoch–Schönlein purpura

- Hyperimmunoglobulinemia D with recurrent fever

- Sarcoidosis

- Whipple's disease

- TNF receptor associated periodic syndrome

- Granulomatosis with polyangiitis (and many other vasculitis syndromes)

- Familial Mediterranean fever

- Systemic lupus erythematosus

An undifferentiated arthritis is an arthritis that does not fit into well-known clinical disease categories, possibly being an early stage of a definite rheumatic disease.

Signs and symptoms of arthritis

Pain, which can vary in severity, is a common symptom in virtually all types of arthritis. Other symptoms include swelling, joint stiffness, redness, and aching around the joint(s). Arthritic disorders like lupus and rheumatoid arthritis can affect other organs in the body, leading to a variety of symptoms.Symptoms may include:

• Inability to use the hand or walk

• Stiffness in one or more joints

• Rash or itch

• Malaise and fatigue

• Weight loss

• Poor sleep

• Muscle aches and pains

• Tenderness

• Difficulty moving the joint

It is common in advanced arthritis for significant secondary changes to occur. For example, arthritic symptoms might make it difficult for a person to move around and/or exercise, which can lead to secondary effects, such as:

• Muscle weakness

• Loss of flexibility

• Decreased aerobic fitness

These changes, in addition to the primary symptoms, can have a huge impact on quality of life.

Disability

Arthritis is the most common cause of disability in the United States. More than 20 million individuals with arthritis have severe limitations in function on a daily basis. Absenteeism and frequent visits to the physician are common in individuals who have arthritis. Arthritis can make it difficult for individuals to be physically active and some become home bound.

It is estimated that the total cost of arthritis cases is close to $100 billion of which almost 50% is from lost earnings. Each year, arthritis results in nearly 1 million hospitalizations and close to 45 million outpatient visits to health care centers.

Decreased mobility, in combination with the above symptoms, can make it difficult for an individual to remain physically active, contributing to an increased risk of obesity, high cholesterol or vulnerability to heart disease. People with arthritis are also at increased risk of depression, which may be a response to numerous factors, including fear of worsening symptoms.

Risk factors

There are common risk factors that increase a person's chance of developing arthritis later in adulthood. Some of these are modifiable while others are not. Smoking has been linked to an increased susceptibility of developing arthritis, particularly rheumatoid arthritis.

What causes arthritis?

Arthritis may be caused byTrusted Source:

• wear and tear of a joint from overuse

• age (OA is most common in adults over age 50)

• injuries

• obesity

• autoimmune disorders

• genes or family history

• muscle weakness

Osteoarthritis

Normal wear and tear cause OA, one of the most common forms of arthritis. An infection or injury to the joints can exacerbate this natural breakdown of cartilage tissue.

Cartilage is a firm but flexible connective tissue in your joints. It protects the joints by absorbing the pressure and shock created when you move and put stress on them. A reduction in the normal amount of this cartilage tissue causes some forms of arthritis.

Rheumatoid arthritis

Another common form of arthritis, RA, is an autoimmune disorder. It occurs when your body's immune system attacks the tissues of the body, resulting in inflammation to joints as well as other body organs.

In the joints, this inflammatory response affects the synovium, a soft tissue in your joints that produces a fluid that nourishes the cartilage and lubricates the joints, eventually destroying both bone and cartilage inside the joint.

The exact cause of the immune system's attacks is unknown. But scientists have discovered genetic markers that increase your risk of developing RA fivefold.

Treatment for Arthritis

There is no known cure for arthritis and rheumatic diseases. Treatment options vary depending on the type of arthritis and include physical therapy, exercise and diet, orthopedic bracing, and oral and topical medications. Joint replacement surgery may be required to repair damage, restore function, or relieve pain.

Physical therapy

In general, studies have shown that physical exercise of the affected joint can noticeably improve long-term pain relief. Furthermore, exercise of the arthritic joint is encouraged to maintain the health of the particular joint and the overall body of the person.

Individuals with arthritis can benefit from both physical and occupational therapy. In arthritis the joints become stiff and the range of movement can be limited. Physical therapy has been shown to significantly improve function, decrease pain, and delay the need for surgical intervention in advanced cases. Exercise prescribed by a physical therapist has been shown to be more effective than medications in treating osteoarthritis of the knee. Exercise often focuses on improving muscle strength, endurance and flexibility. In some cases, exercises may be designed to train balance. Occupational therapy can provide assistance with activities. Assistive technology is a tool used to aid a person's disability by reducing their physical barriers by improving the use of their damaged body part, typically after an amputation. Assistive technology devices can be customized to the patient or bought commercially.

Medications

There are several types of medications that are used for the treatment of arthritis. Treatment typically begins with medications that have the fewest side effects with further medications being added if insufficiently effective.

Depending on the type of arthritis, the medications that are given may be different. For example, the first-line treatment for osteoarthritis is acetaminophen (paracetamol) while for inflammatory arthritis it involves non-steroidal anti-inflammatory drugs (NSAIDs) like ibuprofen. Opioids and NSAIDs may be less well tolerated. However, topical NSAIDs may have better safety profiles than oral NSAIDs. For more severe cases of osteoarthritis, intra-articular corticosteroid injections may also be considered.

The drugs to treat rheumatoid arthritis (RA) range from corticosteroids to monoclonal antibodies given intravenously. Due to the autoimmune nature of RA, treatments may include not only pain medications and anti-inflammatory drugs, but also another category of drugs called disease-modifying antirheumatic drugs (DMARDs). Treatment with DMARDs is designed to slow down the progression of RA by initiating an adaptive immune response, in part by CD4+ T helper (Th) cells, specifically Th17 cells. Th17 cells are present in higher quantities at the site of bone destruction in joints and produce inflammatory cytokines associated with inflammation, such as interleukin-17 (IL-17).

Surgery

A number of rheumasurgical interventions have been incorporated in the treatment of arthritis since the 1950s. Arthroscopic surgery for osteoarthritis of the knee provides no additional benefit to optimized physical and medical therapy.

Adaptive aids

People with hand arthritis can have trouble with simple activities of daily living tasks (ADLs), such as turning a key in a lock or opening jars, as these activities can be cumbersome and painful. There are adaptive aids or assistive devices (ADs) available to help with these tasks, but they are generally more costly than conventional products with the same function. It is now possible to 3-D print adaptive aids, which have been released as open source hardware to reduce patient costs. Adaptive aids can significantly help arthritis patients and the vast majority of those with arthritis need and use them.

Alternative medicine

Further research is required to determine if transcutaneous electrical nerve stimulation (TENS) for knee osteoarthritis is effective for controlling pain.

Low level laser therapy may be considered for relief of pain and stiffness associated with arthritis. Evidence of benefit is tentative.

Pulsed electromagnetic field therapy (PEMFT) has tentative evidence supporting improved functioning but no evidence of improved pain in osteoarthritis. The FDA has not approved PEMFT for the treatment of arthritis. In Canada, PEMF devices are legally licensed by Health Canada for the treatment of pain associated with arthritic conditions.

ARTHRITIS RECIPES

Here, in this part of the book. I made a list of food that are good for people with arthritis and I explained each recipes by listing the ingredients alongside the instructions on how to go about the preparation;

Turmeric Chicken & Quinoa

Equipment

• Dutch Oven

Ingredients

• 2 pounds boneless skinless chicken or tempeh

• 1 teaspoon salt

• ½ teaspoon fresh ground black pepper

• 1 tablespoon extra virgin olive oil

• 1 teaspoon ground turmeric

• 1 onion chopped

• 1 tablespoon grated chopped peeled fresh ginger

- 4 cloves garlic minced

- 2 plum tomatoes chopped

- 1 ½ teaspoon curry powder

- ½ teaspoon ground cumin

- 2 cups quinoa rinsed

- 2 bay leaves

- 1 ½ tablespoons Asian fish sauce

- 2 ¾ cups chicken broth or vegetable broth

Instructions

1. Season the chicken with salt and pepper. In a large Dutch Oven, heat the olive oil to medium and add turmeric. Stir and add chicken.

2. Cook until browned on both sides. Transfer to a plate. Allow to cool and then shred.

3. Add the onion and ginger and cook for 8 minutes. Add garlic, tomatoes, curry powder, cumin and quinoa. Cook, string constantly for 3 minutes.

4. Return the chicken to the pot. Add bay leaves, fish sauce and chicken broth. Bring to a simmer.

5. Cover and cook over low heat for 25 minutes. Remove from heat and let stand covered for 5 minutes.

Gluten-Free Sweet Potato Muffins

Ingredients

• 1 small organic sweet potato, roasted (1 cup, packed)

• 3 organic free-range eggs, lightly beaten

• ¾ cup of organic canned coconut milk

• 2 Tablespoon of organic olive oil

• ½ cup of pure organic maple syrup

• 1 cup of organic brown rice flour

• ¼ cup of organic coconut flour

• 1 Tablespoon baking powder

- ½ teaspoon pink Himalayan salt

- 1 Tablespoon of ground cinnamon

- 1 teaspoon of ground ginger

- ⅛ teaspoon of ground cloves

- ⅛ teaspoon of ground nutmeg

Instructions

1. Preheat oven to 400 degrees Fahrenheit.

2. Oil a 12-hole muffin tray.

3. Poke holes in your sweet potato and place on the middle rack – cook for 60 minutes (or until soft).

4. Remove sweet potato from oven and let cool.

5. Scoop the sweet potato from the skin and place in a mixing bowl.

6. Discard the skin or eat it as a snack – it contains a lot of the same vitamins as the insides!

7. Add olive oil, beaten eggs, coconut milk, and maple syrup to the sweet potato and mix until it is smooth.

8. In a separate bowl, mix the dry ingredients together.

9. Pour the dry ingredients into the sweet potato and mix until well combined.

10. Pour the batter in the muffin pan and fill each tin until ⅔ full.

11. Cook in the oven on the middle rack for 30-35 minutes (or until an inserted knife in the middle of the muffin comes out clean).

12. Now take that muffin and eaaaaaaaaaaat it.

Cherry Mango Anti-Inflammatory Smoothie.

Ingredients

- 1 cup frozen sweet cherries

- ½ cup water

- 1 cup frozen mango

- ¾ cup water

Instructions

1. Place the cherries and mangoes in two separate bowls and let them sit to thaw for about ten minutes.

2. Blend the cherries first: place the cherries and a ½ cup water in the blender and blend on high until smooth. Add the other ¼ cup water if it seems too thick. Pour into a glass.

3. Rinse the blender pitcher and add the mango and the water. Blend on high until smooth. Add more water if needed. Pour into the glass on top of the cherry layer.

4. Enjoy!

Cannellini Beans with Garlic and Sage

Ingredients

Makes about 6 cups

1 pound dried cannellini (white kidney beans)

8 cups room-temperature water

2 tablespoons olive oil

1 large head of garlic, unpeeled, top 1/2 inch cut off to expose cloves

1 large fresh sage sprig

1/4 teaspoon whole black peppercorns

1 teaspoon coarse kosher salt

Extra-virgin olive oil (for drizzling)

Instructions

Step 1

Place beans in large bowl. Cover with cold water (at least 6 cups) and let soak overnight.

Step 2

Drain beans. Place in heavy large pot. Add 8 cups room-temperature water, 2 tablespoons olive oil, garlic, sage, and black peppercorns. Bring to simmer over medium-high heat. Reduce heat to medium-low; simmer uncovered 1 1/2 hours, stirring occasionally. Mix in 1 teaspoon coarse salt. Continue to simmer until beans are tender, adding more water if needed to keep beans covered, about 30 minutes longer. Cool beans in liquid 1 hour.

Step 3

Using slotted spoon, transfer beans to serving bowl, reserving bean cooking liquid, if desired, but discarding garlic, sage, and peppercorns. Season beans to taste with pepper and more coarse salt. Drizzle with extra-virgin olive oil and serve.

Lemon Basil Baked Garlic Butter Salmon

Ingredients

• 6 ounces salmon (4 pieces)

• 2 lemons

• 1/2 cup butter

• 2 Tbs minced garlic

• 1 tsp sweet basil leaf dried

• 1 pinch red pepper flakes more if you like it spicy

• 1 spray PAM cooking spray

Instructions

1. Preheat oven to 375 degrees F.

2. Lay out your foil sheets, one per filet of fish.

3. Put your salmon on your foil.

4. In a microwave safe bowl, combine butter, garlic, basil, and red pepper.

5. Microwave 30 seconds to 1 minute until butter is melted, stir well.

6. Spoon butter mixture evenly over the fish

7. Squeeze half a lemon over each filet

8. Wrap in foil, place on baking sheet

9. Bake for 15-17 minutes, until desired doneness is reached

10. Turn oven on to broil on high

11. Broil 1-2 minutes to crisp up edges of Salmon

12. Serve immediately.

Green Papaya Salad

Ingredients

- ¼ teaspoon freshly grated lime zest

- ¼ cup lime juice

- 2 tablespoons finely chopped palm sugar, or packed brown sugar (see Tip)

- 2 tablespoons fish sauce

- Hawaiian chiles, or any fresh hot chiles, minced, to taste

- 3 cups matchstick-cut or julienned green papaya, (see Tip)

- ½ cup very thinly sliced Maui or other sweet onion

- ½ cup pea shoots, cut into 3-inch pieces, or bean sprouts

- Freshly ground pepper, to taste

Instructions

- Step 1

Whisk lime zest, lime juice, sugar, fish sauce and chiles in a large bowl.

- Step 2

Add papaya, onion and pea shoots (or sprouts) to the vinaigrette; toss to combine. Sprinkle with pepper just before serving.

Lemon Lover's Smoothie

Ingredients

1 lemon large, organic

½ cup coconut milk

½ cup water

0.5 frozen banana

¼ cup raw cashews

1 medjool date

½ tsp vanilla extract

1 tsp lucuma powder optional

handful ice

Instructions

Step 1

Zest your lemon directly into your blender container. Cut away the peel. Then juice the lemon into the bender container, 1 large lemon for a tart smoothie, 1/2 a large or 1 small for a sweet smoothie

Step 2

Add the remaining ingredients and blend until smooth.

Roasted Salmon with Smoky Chickpeas & Greens

Ingredients

- 2 tablespoons extra-virgin olive oil, divided

- 1 tablespoon smoked paprika

- ½ teaspoon salt, divided, plus a pinch

- 1 (15 ounce) can no-salt-added chickpeas, rinsed

- ⅓ cup buttermilk

- ¼ cup mayonnaise

- ¼ cup chopped fresh chives and/or dill, plus more for garnish

- ½ teaspoon ground pepper, divided

- ¼ teaspoon garlic powder

- 10 cups chopped kale

- ¼ cup water

- 1 ¼ pounds wild salmon, cut into 4 portions

Instructions

- Step 1

Position racks in upper third and middle of oven; preheat to 425 degrees F.

- Step 2

Combine 1 tablespoon oil, paprika and 1/4 teaspoon salt in a medium bowl. Very thoroughly pat chickpeas dry, then toss with the paprika mixture. Spread on a rimmed baking sheet. Bake the chickpeas on the upper rack, stirring twice, for 30 minutes.

• Step 3

Meanwhile, puree buttermilk, mayonnaise, herbs, 1/4 teaspoon pepper and garlic powder in a blender until smooth. Set aside.

• Step 4

Heat the remaining 1 tablespoon oil in a large skillet over medium heat. Add kale and cook, stirring occasionally, for 2 minutes. Add water and continue cooking until the kale is tender, about 5 minutes more. Remove from heat and stir in a pinch of salt.

• Step 5

Remove the chickpeas from the oven and push them to one side of the pan. Place salmon on the other side and season with the remaining 1/4 teaspoon each salt and pepper. Bake until the salmon is just cooked through, 5 to 8 minutes.

• Step 6

Drizzle the reserved dressing on the salmon, garnish with more herbs, if desired, and serve with the kale and chickpeas.

Sweet Potato, Kale & Chicken Salad with Peanut Dressing

Ingredients

• 1 pound sweet potatoes (about 2 medium), scrubbed and cut into 1-inch cubes

• 1 ½ teaspoons extra-virgin olive oil

• ¼ teaspoon kosher salt

• ⅛ teaspoon ground pepper

• 1/2 cup Peanut Dressing (see Associated Recipes)

• 6 cups chopped curly kale

• 2 cups shredded cooked chicken breast (see Tip)

• ¼ cup chopped unsalted peanuts

Instructions

- Step 1

Preheat oven to 425 degrees F. Line a rimmed baking sheet with foil; lightly coat with cooking spray. Set aside. Toss sweet potatoes with oil, salt and pepper in a large bowl.

- Step 2

Arrange the sweet potatoes in a single layer on the prepared baking sheet. Roast, turning once, until tender and lightly browned and crispy on the outside, about 20 minutes. Set aside to cool before assembling bowls.

- Step 3

Transfer 2 tablespoons peanut dressing into each of 4 small lidded containers; refrigerate for up to 4 days.

- Step 4

Divide kale among 4 single-serving containers (about 1 1/2 cups each). Top each with one-fourth of the roasted sweet potatoes and 1/2 cup chicken. Seal the containers and refrigerate for up to 4 days.

- Step 5

Just before serving, drizzle each salad with 1 portion of peanut dressing and toss well to coat. Top with 1 tablespoon chopped peanuts.

Herby Mediterranean Fish with Wilted Greens & Mushrooms

Ingredients

- 3 tablespoons olive oil, divided

- ½ large sweet onion, sliced

- 3 cups sliced cremini mushrooms

- 2 cloves garlic, sliced

- 4 cups chopped kale

- 1 medium tomato, diced

- 2 teaspoons Mediterranean Herb Mix (see Associated Recipes), divided

- 1 tablespoon lemon juice

- ½ teaspoon salt, divided

- ½ teaspoon ground pepper, divided

- 4 (4 ounce) cod, sole, or tilapia fillets

- Chopped fresh parsley, for garnish

Instructions

- Step 1

Heat 1 Tbsp. oil in a large saucepan over medium heat. Add onion; cook, stirring occasionally, until translucent, 3 to 4 minutes. Add mushrooms and garlic; cook, stirring occasionally, until the mushrooms release their liquid and begin to brown, 4 to 6 minutes. Add kale, tomato, and 1 tsp. herb mix. Cook, stirring occasionally, until the kale is wilted and the mushrooms are tender, 5 to 7 minutes. Stir in lemon juice and 1/4 tsp. each salt and pepper. Remove from heat, cover, and keep warm.

- Step 2

Sprinkle fish with the remaining 1 tsp. herb mix and 1/4 tsp. each salt and pepper. Heat the remaining 2

Tbsp. oil in a large nonstick skillet over medium-high heat. Add the fish and cook until the flesh is opaque, 2 to 4 minutes per side, depending on thickness. Transfer the fish to 4 plates or a serving platter. Top and surround the fish with the vegetables; sprinkle with parsley, if desired.

Orange Creamsicle Chia Pudding

Ingredients

• 2 tbsp chia seeds

• 1/4 scoop vanilla protein powder vegan

• 1 mandarin orange

• honey to taste

• 3/4 cup oat milk

Instructions

1. Add the chia seeds, oat milk, protein powder, and honey to a bowl.

2. Stir the bowl until the ingredients are mixed together.

3. Place the bowl in the refrigerator for about 30 minutes or until a "chia pudding" forms.

4. Remove from refrigerator and top with fresh mandarin slices.

White Bean & Veggie Salad

Ingredients

- 2 cups mixed salad greens

- ¾ cup veggies of your choice, such as chopped cucumbers and cherry tomatoes

- ⅓ cup canned white beans, rinsed and drained

- ½ avocado, diced

- 1 tablespoon red-wine vinegar

- 2 teaspoons extra-virgin olive oil

- ¼ teaspoon kosher salt

- Freshly ground pepper to taste

Instructions

- Step 1

Combine greens, veggies, beans and avocado in a medium bowl. Drizzle with vinegar and oil and season with salt and pepper. Toss to combine and transfer to a large plate.

Blueberry Almond Chia Pudding

Ingredients

- ½ cup unsweetened almond milk or other nondairy milk beverage

- 2 tablespoons chia seeds

- 2 teaspoons pure maple syrup

- ⅛ teaspoon almond extract

- ½ cup fresh blueberries, divided

- 1 tablespoon toasted slivered almonds, divided

Instructions

- Step 1

Stir together almond milk (or other nondairy milk beverage), chia, maple syrup and almond extract in a small bowl. Cover and refrigerate for at least 8 hours and up to 3 days.

- Step 2

When ready to serve, stir the pudding well. Spoon about half the pudding into a serving glass (or bowl) and top with half the blueberries and almonds. Add the rest of the pudding and top with the remaining blueberries and almonds.

Greek Roasted Fish with Vegetables

Ingredients

- 1 pound fingerling potatoes, halved lengthwise

- 2 tablespoons olive oil

- 5 garlic cloves, coarsely chopped

- ½ teaspoon sea salt

- ½ teaspoon freshly ground black pepper

- 4 5 to 6-ounce fresh or frozen skinless salmon fillets

- 2 medium red, yellow and/or orange sweet peppers, cut into rings

- 2 cups cherry tomatoes

- 1 ½ cups chopped fresh parsley (1 bunch)

- ¼ cup pitted kalamata olives, halved

- ¼ cup finely snipped fresh oregano or 1 Tbsp. dried oregano, crushed

- 1 lemon

Instructions

- Step 1

Preheat oven to 425 degrees F. Place potatoes in a large bowl. Drizzle with 1 Tbsp. of the oil and sprinkle with garlic and 1/8 tsp. of the salt and black pepper; toss to coat. Transfer to a 15x10-inch baking pan; cover with foil. Roast 30 minutes.

- Step 2

Meanwhile, thaw salmon, if frozen. Combine, in the same bowl, sweet peppers, tomatoes, parsley, olives, oregano and 1/8 tsp. of the salt and black pepper. Drizzle with remaining 1 Tbsp. oil; toss to coat.

- Step 3

Rinse salmon; pat dry. Sprinkle with remaining 1/4 tsp. salt and black pepper. Spoon sweet pepper mixture over potatoes and top with salmon. Roast, uncovered, 10 minutes more or just until salmon flakes.

- Step 4

Remove zest from lemon. Squeeze juice from lemon over salmon and vegetables. Sprinkle with zest.

Vegan Coconut Chickpea Curry

Ingredients

- 2 teaspoons avocado oil or canola oil

- 1 cup chopped onion

- 1 cup diced bell pepper

- 1 medium zucchini, halved and sliced

- 1 (15 ounce) can chickpeas, drained and rinsed

- 1 ½ cups coconut curry simmer sauce (see Tip)

- ½ cup vegetable broth

- 4 cups baby spinach

- 2 cups precooked brown rice, heated according to package instructions

Instructions

- Step 1

Heat oil in a large skillet over medium-high heat. Add onion, pepper and zucchini; cook, stirring often, until the vegetables begin to brown, 5 to 6 minutes.

- Step 2

Add chickpeas, simmer sauce and broth and bring to a simmer, stirring. Reduce heat to medium-low and simmer until the vegetables are tender, 4 to 6 minutes. Stir in spinach just before serving. Serve over rice.

Creamy Chicken, Brussels Sprouts & Mushrooms One-Pot Pasta

Ingredients

- 8 ounces whole-wheat linguine or spaghetti

- 1 pound boneless, skinless chicken thighs

- 4 cups sliced mushrooms

- 2 cups sliced Brussels sprouts

- 1 medium onion, chopped

- 4 cloves garlic, thinly sliced

- 2 tablespoons Boursin cheese

- 1 ¼ teaspoons dried thyme

- ¾ teaspoon dried rosemary

- ¾ teaspoon salt

- 4 cups water

- 2 tablespoons chopped fresh chives

Instructions

- Step 1

Combine pasta, chicken, mushrooms, Brussels sprouts, onion, garlic, Boursin cheese, thyme, rosemary and salt in a large pot. Stir in water. Bring to a boil over high heat. Boil, stirring frequently, until the pasta is cooked and the water has almost evaporated, 10 to 12 minutes. Remove from heat and let stand, stirring occasionally, for 5 minutes. Serve sprinkled with chives.

Mediterranean Breakfast Sandwiches

Ingredients

- 4 multigrain sandwich thins

- 4 teaspoons olive oil

- 1 tablespoon snipped fresh rosemary or 1/2 teaspoon dried rosemary, crushed

- 4 eggs

- 2 cups fresh baby spinach leaves

- 1 medium tomato, cut into 8 thin slices

- 4 tablespoons reduced-fat feta cheese

- ⅛ teaspoon kosher salt

- Freshly ground black pepper

Instructions

- Step 1

Preheat oven to 375 degrees F. Split sandwich thins; brush cut sides with 2 teaspoons of the olive oil. Place on baking sheet; toast in oven about 5 minutes or until edges are light brown and crisp.

- Step 2

Meanwhile, in a large skillet heat the remaining 2 teaspoons olive oil and the rosemary over medium-high heat. Break eggs, one at a time, into skillet. Cook about 1 minute or until whites are set but yolks are still runny. Break yolks with spatula. Flip eggs; cook on other side until done. Remove from heat.

- Step 3

Place the bottom halves of the toasted sandwich thins on four serving plates. Divide spinach among sandwich thins on plates. Top each with two of the tomato slices, an egg and 1 tablespoon of the feta cheese. Sprinkle with the salt and pepper. Top with the remaining sandwich thin halves.

Smoky Spanish-Style Chicken With Patatas Bravas

Ingredients

For 2 people [double for 4]

2 British chicken breast portions

4 white potatoes

50ml mayonnaise †

16g tomato paste

1/2 tsp dried chilli flakes

2 tsp ground coriander

2 tsp smoked paprika

1 red onion

1 red pepper

1 garlic clove

1 tomato

1 yellow pepper

Pepper, salt, sugar, vegetable oil

Instructions

For 2 people [double for 4]

1. Before you start cooking, take your chicken out of the fridge, open the packet and let it air, then preheat the oven to 220°C/ 200°C (fan)/ gas 6

Cut the potatoes (skins on) into bite-sized cubes, then add them to a baking tray with a drizzle of vegetable oil and a pinch of salt and pepper

Put the tray in the oven for 25-30 min or until the potatoes are golden and crispy – these are your crispy potatoes

2. Deseed the peppers (scrape the seeds and pith out with a teaspoon) and cut them into thick strips

Peel and roughly slice the red onion[s]

Add the pepper strips and sliced onion to a separate baking tray with a drizzle of vegetable oil and a pinch of salt

Put the tray in the oven for 20 min or until the veg is soft and tender

3. While the veg is in the oven, boil half a kettle

Dice the tomato[es]

Peel and finely chop (or grate) the garlic

Dissolve the tomato paste in 100ml [200ml] boiled water and add the chilli flakes (can't handle the heat? Go easy!) – this is your spicy tomato stock

4. Heat a large, wide-based pan (preferably non-stick) with a drizzle of vegetable oil over a medium heat

Once hot, add the diced tomato with a pinch of salt and sugar and cook for 3-4 min or until the tomatoes have broken down

Add the spicy tomato stock to the pan and cook for 3-4 min further or until thickened – this is your bravas sauce

5. While the sauce thickens, cut the chicken breast portions in half lengthways

Combine the ground coriander, smoked paprika, 1 tsp [2 tsp] sugar and a generous pinch of salt on a plate – this is your smoky spice mix

Add the halved chicken breasts to the smoky spice mix and mix until they are fully coated – this is your coated chicken

6. Heat a separate large, wide-based pan (preferably non-stick) with a drizzle of vegetable oil over a medium heat

Once hot, add the coated chicken and cook for 4-5 min on each side or until the chicken is slightly blackened on the outside and cooked through (no pink meat!) – this is your smoky Spanish-style chicken

7. Meanwhile, combine the mayo, chopped garlic, 1 tsp [2 tsp] cold water and a pinch of salt in a small bowl – this is your aioli

To serve, top the roasted veg with the smoky Spanish-style chicken with the crispy potatoes to the side

Spoon the bravas sauce over the crispy potatoes – this is your patatas bravas

Drizzle the aioli all over the patatas bravas

Enjoy!

Citrus Vinaigrette

Ingredients

- ½ small shallot, quartered

- 1 teaspoon orange zest

- ¼ cup orange juice, preferably freshly squeezed

- 2 tablespoons lemon juice

- 2 teaspoons Dijon mustard

- ½ teaspoon salt

- ½ teaspoon ground pepper

- ¼ cup extra-virgin olive oil

- ¼ cup organic canola oil or avocado oil

Instructions

- Step 1

Combine shallot, orange zest, orange juice, lemon juice, mustard, salt and pepper in a blender or mini food processor. (Alternatively, combine in a jar and use an immersion blender.) Add olive oil and canola (or avocado) oil; blend until smooth.

Kale & Avocado Salad with Blueberries & Edamame

Ingredients

- 6 cups stemmed and coarsely chopped curly kale

- 1 avocado, diced

- 1 cup blueberries

- 1 cup halved yellow cherry tomatoes

- 1 cup cooked shelled edamame

- ¼ cup sliced almonds, toasted

- ½ cup crumbled goat cheese (2 ounces)

- ¼ cup olive oil

- 3 tablespoons lemon juice

- 1 tablespoon minced chives

- 1 ½ teaspoons honey

- 1 teaspoon Dijon mustard

- 1 teaspoon salt

Instructions

- Step 1

Place kale in a large bowl and, using your hands, massage to soften the leaves. Add avocado, blueberries, tomatoes, edamame, almonds, and goat cheese.

- Step 2

Combine oil, lemon juice, chives, honey, mustard, and salt in a small bowl or in a jar with a tight-fitting lid. Whisk or shake well.

- Step 3

Drizzle the vinaigrette over the salad and toss to combine.

Hummus & Greek Salad

Ingredients

- 2 cups arugula

- ⅓ cup cherry tomatoes, halved

- ⅓ cup sliced cucumber

- 1 tablespoon chopped red onion

- 1 ½ tablespoons extra-virgin olive oil

- 2 teaspoons red-wine vinegar

- ⅛ teaspoon ground pepper

- 1 tablespoon feta cheese

- 1 4-inch whole-wheat pita

- ¼ cup hummus

Instructions

- Step 1

Toss arugula in a bowl with tomatoes, cucumber, onion, oil, vinegar and pepper. Top with feta. Serve with pita and hummus.

Antiinflammatory Salads (cold and warm)

Ingredients

Dressing

olive oil

turmeric

ginger

lemon juice

garlic

dijon mustard

Cold Salad

kale

pecans

red onion

mint

Warm Salad

broccoli

cauliflower

brussels sprouts

carrots

parsley

shallots

Instructions

Dressing

Step 1

Add to blender and blend until smooth.

Cold Salad

Step 1

Chop kale.

Step 2

Add rest of ingredients.

Step 3

Add dressing.

Step 4

Massage kale.

Warm Salad

Step 1

Toss vegetables with olive oil, salt and pepper.

Step 2

Roast 350F for 10 minutes.

Step 3

Drizzle with dressing.

Feel-good pineapple smoothie

Ingredients

• 1 ½ cups frozen pineapple chunks

• 1 orange, peeled

• 1 cup coconut water

• 1 tablespoon finely-chopped fresh ginger (or 1/4 teaspoon ground ginger)

• 1 teaspoon chia seeds, plus extra for garnishing

• 1 teaspoon McCormick Ground Turmeric

• 1/4 teaspoon ground black pepper

Instructions

1. Add all ingredients to a blender. Pulse until smooth.

2. Serve immediately, garnished with extra chia seeds if desired.

Peanut Zucchini Noodle Salad with Chicken

Ingredients

- ¾ cup creamy natural peanut butter

- ¾ cup hot water

- ¼ cup lime juice

- 2 tablespoons light brown sugar

- 2 tablespoons reduced-sodium tamari or soy sauce

- 1 ½ tablespoons fish sauce

- 1 teaspoon hot sauce, such as Sriracha

- 1 teaspoon grated garlic

- 4 cups spiralized zucchini (1 large)

- 3 cups spiralized red cabbage (about 1/2 small head)

- 1 cup spiralized carrot (1 large)

- ½ cup chopped fresh cilantro

- 2 cups shredded rotisserie chicken (8 ounces)

- ¼ cup chopped unsalted roasted peanuts

Instructions

- Step 1

Combine peanut butter, water, lime juice, brown sugar, tamari (or soy sauce), fish sauce, hot sauce and garlic in a blender. Pulse until smooth.

- Step 2

Combine zucchini, cabbage, carrot and cilantro in a large bowl. Add 1 cup of the dressing (reserve the rest for another use) and toss to coat. Top the salad with chicken and peanuts. Serve immediately.

Anti-inflammatory beet & cherry smoothie

Ingredients

1. 10 oz of unsweetened vanilla almond milk

2. 1-2 small beets, cut into quarters (store bought, already peeled and ready to eat)

3. 1/2 cup of frozen pitted cherries

4. 1/2 frozen banana

5. 1 tablespoon of almonds/almond butter

Instructions

1. add all ingredients to a high speed blender and blend until smooth.

5 Ingredient Thai Pumpkin Soup

Ingredients

• 2 tablespoons red curry paste

• 4 cups chicken or vegetable broth , about 32 ounces

• 2 15 ounce cans pumpkin puree

• 1 3/4 cup coconut milk , or a 13.5 ounce can, reserving 1 tablespoon

• 1 large red chili pepper , sliced

• cilantro for garnish if desired

Instructions

1. In a large saucepan over medium heat, cook the curry paste for about one minute or until paste becomes fragrant. Add the broth and the pumpkin and stir.

2. Cook for about 3 minutes or until soup starts to bubble. Add the coconut milk and cook until hot, about 3 minutes.

3. Ladle into bowls and garnish with a drizzle of the reserved coconut milk and sliced red chilis. Garnish with cilantro leaves if desired.

Apple And Ginger Smoothie

Ingredients:

o 1 ½ cup of fresh pineapples

o One whole banana (it will help reduce the acidity of the drink) o ½ cup of Yogurt (the lactic acid will provide as a soothing agent)

o 1 Tbsp fresh Ginger

o Pinch of ground cinnamon

o 1 tsp turmeric

o Water or pineapple juice as required to keep the consistency of the smoothie medium.

Instructions

Blend all the ingredients in a blender until they blend into a smooth paste. Add cinnamon as a garnish. Serve immediately. Add some ice to take the bite-off the drink and make it more palatable. You can enjoy this drink once every alternate day to detoxify your body of all the toxins and get freedom from pain and inflammation.

Green Salad with Edamame & Beets

Ingredients

• 2 cups mixed salad greens

- 1 cup shelled edamame, thawed

- ½ medium raw beet, peeled and shredded (about 1/2 cup)

- 1 tablespoon plus 1 1/2 teaspoons red-wine vinegar

- 1 tablespoon chopped fresh cilantro

- 2 teaspoons extra-virgin olive oil

- Freshly ground pepper to taste

Instructions

- Step 1

Arrange greens, edamame and beet on a large plate. Whisk vinegar, cilantro, oil, salt and pepper in a small bowl. Drizzle over the salad and enjoy.

Broccoli Stalk Soup

Ingredients

2 broccoli stems

chopped

1 broccoli crown

small, broken into florets

1 carrot

chopped

½ tsp salt

water

to cover veggies

½ cup sunflower seeds

or cashews, soaked for a couple of hours

Instructions

Step 1

Put the broccoli stalks, florets, carrots and salt in a medium sized pot. Add just enough water so the vegetables are barely covered.

Step 2

Bring to a boil. Lower the heat, cover, and simmer for 20 minutes.

Step 3

Drain the sunflower seeds or cashews and rinse them well.

Step 4

Add everything into a blender and blend until smooth. Taste and adjust seasoning if necessary.

CONCLUSION

Since arthritis means inflammation, it's essential to tune down the latter. So, before you start looking for the right pills to ease the pain, see what some homemade fusions can do for you. The recipes for regular and rheumatoid arthritis, as well as for gout, must always include at least one anti-inflammatory ingredient, such as turmeric, ginger, pineapples, different kinds of berries, especially strawberries and cherries, mango, kiwi and more.

If you had enough of the joint stiffness and constant swelling, give these arthritis reversal smoothies a shot. You won't need anything special, just blend the ingredients together until there are no lumps, then add some water (as per the recipe), give them a little stir and drink up!